PRE- AND POSTANESTHESIA NURSING
KNOWLEDGE BASE AND
CLINICAL COMPETENCIES

PRE- AND POSTANESTHESIA NURSING KNOWLEDGE BASE AND CLINICAL COMPETENCIES

Maria T. Zickuhr, MSN, RN, CPAN

Formerly Nurse Manager
Post Anesthesia Care Unit
Pre Care and TCI Center
The Cleveland Clinic Foundation
Cleveland, Ohio

Deborah Brown Atsberger, MSN, RN, CPAN

Clinical Instructor for the Post Anesthesia Care Unit
The Cleveland Clinic Foundation
Cleveland, Ohio

W. B. SAUNDERS COMPANY
A Division of Harcourt Brace & Company
Philadelphia, London, Toronto, Montreal, Sydney, Tokyo

W. B. SAUNDERS COMPANY

A Division of Harcourt Brace & Company

The Curtis Center
Independence Square West
Philadelphia, Pennsylvania 19106

Library of Congress Cataloging-in-Publication Data

Zickuhr, Maria T.
    Pre- and postanesthesia nursing knowledge base and clinical
competencies / Maria T. Zickuhr, Deborah Brown Atsberger.
        p.   cm.
    Includes bibliographical references.
    ISBN 0-7216-5645-5
    1. Post anesthesia nursing.   2. Preanesthetic medication.
3. Preoperative care.   I. Zickuhr, Maria T.   II. Title.
    [DNLM: 1. Postanesthesia Nursing—standards.   2. Preoperative
Care—standards.   WY 154 A882p 1995]
RD51.3.A88   1995
610.73'677—dc20
DNLM/DLC   94-25911

Pre- and Postanesthesia Nursing Knowledge Base and Clinical Competencies

Copyright © 1995 by W. B. Saunders Company.   ISBN 0-7216-5645-5

Printed in the United States of America

Last digit is the print number: 9   8   7   6   5   4   3   2   1

Acknowledgment

In 1983, a group of staff nurses were convened to develop behavioral objectives for postanesthesia care. The behavioral objectives were then organized into levels of postanesthesia nursing practice. The initial format for the levels of practice was developed by Deborah Atsberger, Clinical Instructor and Maria Zickuhr, together with the rest of the management team, Melissa Magdinec, Susan Rutledge, Susan Simon, compiled the objectives and edited the product.

In 1987, the Pediatric Clinical Competencies were developed for both the pre- and postanesthesia nurses. Deborah Atsberger spearheaded the endeavor together with Susan Rutledge, Joy Markel, Maria Zickuhr and the Pediatric Pre and Post-anesthesia Staff Nurses.

In 1989, the Preanesthesia Levels of Practice were developed by Joy Markel, Deborah Atsberger, Maria Zickuhr, together with the Preanesthesia Staff Nurses and was expanded to four levels of practice in 1993.

In 1992, the Postanesthesia Knowledge Base and Clinical Competencies, were revised by Diane Arpey and Mary Markiewitz.

These knowledge-based objectives and nursing care competencies have grown as the speciality of pre- and postanesthesia nursing has grown. The numerous pre- and postanesthesia nurses at the Cleveland Clinic Foundation who have participated in the development, implementation, evaluation and revision of the objectives and competencies are acknowledged for their commitment to the specialty of pre- and postanesthesia nursing.

Contents

1

General Introduction

These knowledge-based objectives and nursing care competencies were developed by the Pre- and Post Anesthesia Care Unit (PACU) of The Cleveland Clinic Foundation. They are intended to be used as flexible guidelines, and will continue to grow and develop as the specialty of postanesthesia nursing grows and develops. Statements within each level are based on assumptions that all previous levels have been obtained.

These objectives and competencies are not totally inclusive statements of nursing practice. They are to be used with hospital policy, procedures, and job descriptions in conjunction with the basic standard for professional practice. In order to provide competent professional postanesthesia nursing care, the nurse must be able to treat patients with dignity and concern, demonstrate compassion for patients, be willing to give psychological support, maintain satisfactory working relationships, and communicate and cooperate effectively.

Purpose

The purpose of the knowledge-based objectives and the nursing care competencies is multifold:

1. To provide a standard for safe pre- and postanesthesia nursing practice.
2. To direct the activity of nursing knowledge and skill specific to pre- and postanesthesia care.
3. To direct the individual nurse toward a professional practice by providing guidelines for pacing the acquisition of knowledge, thereby taking a joint responsibility in his/her own development.
4. To direct the clinical instructor in providing adequate orientation and ongoing inservice.
5. To provide the nurse managers with guidelines for performance appraisals.
6. To provide the pre- and postanesthesia nurse with guidelines for his/her own self-evaluations, thereby making the evaluation process a joint effort.

Levels of Nursing Practice for Pre- and Post Anesthesia Nursing

Level I	Level II	Level III	Level IV
Beginner Pre- & Post Anesthesia Nurse	**Pre- & Post Anesthesia Nurse**	**Senior Pre- & Post Anesthesia Nurse**	**Advanced Pre- & Post Anesthesia Nurse**
Step 1/Step 2 General practitioner; needs direct supervision in pre- postanesthesia nursing Identifies and evaluates nursing interventions with assistance	Beginner charge and teacher 1:1; needs general supervision Identifies and evaluates nursing interventions	Experienced charge and teacher 1:1; needs little supervision Manages and coordinates nursing staff for a specific shift	Step 1/Step 2 Manager of patient care, nursing administration; researcher Participates in unit development

PART ONE

POST ANESTHESIA NURSING KNOWLEDGE BASE AND CLINICAL COMPETENCIES

Definition of Postanesthesia Nursing

Postanesthesia nursing is an area of professional nursing practice that renders acute care by specially educated nursing personnel who have the ability to recognize and manage the problems particular to patients emerging from drug-induced coma, sympathetic blockade, or nerve block.

Framework for Postanesthesia Nursing Knowledge Base and Clinical Competencies

I. Provides Nursing Care to Patients with Alterations in Health Management

II. Provides Nursing Care to Patients with Alterations in Activity-Exercise Patterns

III. Provides Nursing Care to Patients with Alterations in Cognitive and Perceptual Patterns

IV. Participates in Professional Growth and Development

2

Beginner
Post Anesthesia Nurse

Level I/Step 1

I. Provides Nursing Care to Patients with Alterations in Health Management

    A. Demonstrates competency in caring for noncomplex postanesthesia patients

    B. Provides for the physical safety of patients

    C. Provides for the communication of health data

II. Provides Nursing Care to Patients with Alterations in Activity-Exercise Patterns

    A. With direction, provides nursing care to patients with potential for respiratory dysfunction

    B. With direction, provides nursing care to patients with artificial airways

    C. With direction, provides nursing care to patients with potential for alterations in cardiac output

III. Provides Nursing Care to Patients with Alterations in Cognitive and Perceptual Patterns

    A. With direction, provides nursing care to patients with alterations in level of consciousness

    B. With direction, provides nursing care to patients with impaired mobility

IV. Participates in Professional Growth and Development

    A. Takes initiative in own professional growth

Postanesthesia Nursing Knowledge Level I/Step 1	Comments/Goals	Competency Met Date and Initial
I. Provides Nursing Care to Patients with Alterations in Health Management		
1. Discusses their interpretation of the various aspects of the postanesthesia nursing care standard		
2. States the normal vital sign parameters		
3. Lists special needs and nursing care of patients undergoing surgical procedures, as written in the Standards of Nursing Care Manual		
4. Identifies other forms of reference when presented with diverse surgical patients		
5. Describes the postanesthesia scoring system		
6. Discusses the requirements for patient discharge		
7. Lists three reasons IV fluids are kept away from the head of the bed		

Postanesthesia Nursing Knowledge *Continued* Level I/Step 1	Comments/Goals	Competency Met Date and Initial
8. Discusses four safety measures pertinent to post-anesthesia care		
9. Lists reasons for the additional steroid doses given perioperatively		
10. Lists three commonly used steroids, their duration and two side effects		
II. Provides Nursing Care to Patients with Alterations in Activity-Exercise Patterns		
1. Describes normal and abnormal breath sounds		
2. Differentiates between oral and nasal airways, and endotracheal and tracheal airways		
3. Discusses the signs and sounds of impending or actual respiratory distress		

Continued on following page.

Postanesthesia Nursing Knowledge *Continued* Level I/Step 1	Comments/Goals	Competency Met Date and Initial
4. Indicates interventions that prevent respiratory distress		
5. Describes nursing responsibilities for patients on ventilators		
6. Calculates correct patient tidal volumes and vital capacities		
7. Defines negative inspiratory force		
8. Lists criteria for each step of the respiratory support weaning process, including extubation		
9. States PACU protocol governing who extubates, and the amount of time the patient is required to stay in PACU after extubation and nursing care following extubation		
10. Discusses respiratory care procedures, as described in the Respiratory Care Study Guide		

Continued on following page.

Postanesthesia Nursing Knowledge *Continued* Level I/Step 1	Comments/Goals	Competency Met Date and Initial
11. Describes bronchopulmonary hygiene techniques		
12. Describes appropriate IV therapy in the postanesthesia setting		
13. Discusses the importance of central venous pressure readings and of correct central venous catheter placement, and states normal readings		
14. States signs and symptoms of hypovolemic shock and explains nursing interventions and medical treatment for prevention		
15. Identifies cardiac arrhythmias		
16. Lists actions, dosage, and one side effect of atropine, lidocaine, propranolol, labetalol, phenylephrine, ephedrine, and hydralazine		
17. Describes expected vascular assessment related to the type of surgery		

Continued on following page

Postanesthesia Nursing Knowledge *Continued* Level I/Step 1	Comments/Goals	Competency Met Date and Initial
III. Provides Nursing Care to Patients with Alterations in Cognitive and Perceptual Patterns		
1. Defines general anesthesia and regional anesthesia		
2. States who is responsible for the sedation and pain relief of postanesthesia patients, and states the PACU protocol		
3. Lists five common narcotics and two sedatives used in the postanesthesia period, discussing expected duration of action, dosage, and two side effects		
4. Discusses the dosage and correct administration of reversal agents; naloxone and physostigmine; states one side effect of each		
5. Lists four commonly used inhalation agents and one side effect, as discussed in the PACU orientation		
6. Lists action, onset, duration and recovery period of propofol (Diprivan)		
7. States the reflexes that return as the patient emerges from general anesthesia		

Continued on following page

Postanesthesia Nursing Knowledge *Continued* Level I/Step 1	Comments/Goals	Competency Met Date and Initial
8. States action, dosage, and duration of droperidol (Inapsine)		
9. Names the dissociative anesthesia agent and lists postanesthesia nursing precautions		
10. Describes components of neurologic assessments		
11. Describes neuromuscular blockade; lists signs of reversal		
12. Lists two common neuromuscular blocking agents, their normal dosages, and duration of action		
13. Lists one common neuromuscular blocking reversal agent, its normal dosage, duration of effect, and common side effect		
14. Defines four different types of regional anesthesia and lists their major postanesthesia complications		

Continued on following page

Postanesthesia Nursing Knowledge *Continued* Level I/Step 1	Comments/Goals	Competency Met Date and Initial
15. Locates three pertinent dermatome levels		
16. Lists the criteria for discharge of patients having had regional anesthesia		

Postanesthesia Nursing Competencies *Continued* Level I/Step 1	Comments/Goals	Competency Met Date and Initial
I. Provides Nursing Care to Patients with Alterations in Health Management		
A. Demonstrates Competency in Caring for Noncomplex Postanesthesia Patients		
1. Initiates the PACU admission procedures:		
a. Includes necessary assessments		
b. Identifies variances from the normal vital sign parameters		
2. Completes admission assessment in a timely manner		
3. Utilizes postanesthesia scoring system		
4. Implements appropriate nursing interventions under direct supervision:		

Continued on following page

Postanesthesia Nursing Competencies *Continued* Level I/Step 1	Comments/Goals	Competency Met Date and Initial
a. Utilizes Standards of Care Manual		
b. Initiates the stir-up regimen		
c. Initiates physician orders		
5. Utilizes the proper reference material before implementing nursing interventions for unfamiliar surgeries or procedures		
6. Sets priorities on own patient case load		
7. Identifies patients who meet the PACU discharge criteria		
8. Promptly discharges patients		

Continued on following page

Postanesthesia Nursing Competencies *Continued* Level I/Step 1	Comments/Goals	Competency Met Date and Initial
9. Knowledgeably administers steroids		
B. Provides for the Physical Safety of Patients		
1. Keeps IV fluids away from the head of the bed		
2. Sets up, uses, and properly cares for equipment (see equipment checklist)		
3. Maintains side rails and crib rails in up position		
4. Prevent injury with use of padding and/or soft restraints		
5. Describes fire safety (see checklist)		
6. Describes triple-page procedure (code blue)		

Continued on following page

Postanesthesia Nursing Competencies *Continued* Level I/Step 1	Comments/Goals	Competency Met Date and Initial
C. Provides for the Communication of Health Data		
1. Obtains health data from anesthesia report, physical assessment, and review of records		
2. Documents pertinent health data		
3. Documents the admission and on-going physical assessments using anatomical landmarks (includes all aspects according to the PACU standard of care)		
4. Documents the plan of care		
5. Keeps nurse coordinator informed of patient status		
6. Identifies medical and surgical services involved in individual patient's care		
7. Gives accurate patient reports		

Continued on following page

Postanesthesia Nursing Competencies *Continued* Level I/Step 1	Comments/Goals	Competency Met Date and Initial
8. Completes the Postanesthesia Nursing Condition Report		
9. Writes a discharge summary incorporating unresolved nursing diagnoses		

Postanesthesia Nursing Competencies *Continued* Level 1/Step 1	Comments/Goals	Competency Met Date and Initial
II. Provides Nursing Care to Patients with Alterations in Activity-Exercise Pattern		
A. With Direction, Provides Nursing Care to Patients with Potential for Respiratory Dysfunction		
1. Correctly auscultates breath sounds and checks for adequacy of ventilatory volumes		
2. Distinguish between normal and abnormal breath sounds		
3. Obtains arterial blood gas samples from arterial line		
4. Identifies the sights and sounds of:		
a. Airway obstruction		
b. Laryngospasm		
c. Bronchospasm		

Continued on following page

Postanesthesia Nursing Competencies *Continued* Level I/Step 1	Comments/Goals	Competency Met Date and Initial
d. Aspiration		
e. Respiratory arrest		
5. Initiates nursing intervention to provide for the first steps in treating the above distress:		
a. Positioning		
b. Oral/nasal suctioning		
c. Insertion of oral/nasal airways		
d. Bag/mask ventilation		

Continued on following page

Postanesthesia Nursing Competencies *Continued* Level I/Step 1	Comments/Goals	Competency Met Date and Initial
6. Initiates effective bronchopulmonary hygiene		
B. With Direction, Provides Nursing Care to Patients with Artificial Airways		
1. Maintains airway patency:		
a. Performs proper tracheostomy care		
b. Hyperventilates and suctions endotracheal tube		
c. Maintains cuff pressures		
2. Initiates nursing responsibilities for patient on ventilator		
3. Checks ventilator prior to patient use		

Continued on following page

Postanesthesia Nursing Competencies *Continued* Level I/Step 1	Comments/Goals	Competency Met Date and Initial
4. Applies ventilator to patient with normal ventilator status		
5. Weans patient from Bird/Servo ventilator		
6. Identifies person responsible for extubation		
C. With Direction, Provides Nursing Care to Patients with Potential for Alterations in Cardiac Output		
1. Identifies normal blood pressure ranges		
2. Identifies sinus rhythm, PVC, PAC, bradycardia, tachycardia, junctional rhythm, atrial fibrillation, atrial flutter, ventricular tachycardia, and ventricular fibrillation.		
3. Initiates appropriate peripheral vascular assessments		

Postanesthesia Nursing Competencies *Continued* Level I/Step 1	Comments/Goals	Competency Met Date and Initial
4. Differentiates between IV therapy for pediatric, geriatric, adult, and high-risk patients		
5. Assesses fluid status, IV sites, and time tapes on IV bottles/bags		
6. Identifies deviations from the normal CVP readings		
7. Identifies correct central venous catheter placement		
8. Performs accurate CVP readings		
9. Identifies normal arterial waveform and maintains arterial line patency		
10. Documents accurate intake and output		

Continued on following page

Postanesthesia Nursing Competencies *Continued* Level I/Step 1	Comments/Goals	Competency Met Date and Initial
11. Applies cardiac monitor; sets alarms and parameters appropriately		
12. Runs a 12-lead EKG with rhythm strip		
13. Lists symptoms, nursing interventions, and expected medical interventions for hypovolemic shock		
14. Initiates immediate nursing interventions for the treatment of hypotension, arrhythmias, and cardiac arrest:		
a. Positions patient appropriately		
b. Administers lidocaine, atropine, and propranolol correctly		
c. Demonstrates effective cardiac compressions		

Postanesthesia Nursing Competencies *Continued* Level I/Step 1	Comments/Goals	Competency Met Date and Initial
III. Provides Nursing Care to Patients with Alterations in Cognitive and Perceptual Patterns		
A. With Direction, Provides Nursing Care to Patients with Alterations in Level of Consciousness		
1. Differentiates between types of anesthesia		
2. Knowledgeably administers narcotics, sedatives, and their reversal agents:		
a. Follows the PACU protocol for patient sedation and pain relief		
b. Refers to appropriate physician for postanesthesia pain management		
c. Administers common agents correctly		
3. Identifies postanesthesia patients who need additional precautions before administering narcotics		
4. Identifies three commonly used inhalation agents		

Continued on following page

Postanesthesia Nursing Competencies *Continued* Level I/Step 1	Comments/Goals	Competency Met Date and Initial
5. Initiates postanesthesia nursing precautions for patients who have had a dissociative anesthesia agent		
6. Identifies on admission and throughout recovery the patient's level of consciousness		
7. Monitors the progression of the patient's postanesthesia recovery		
8. Initiates appropriate neurological assessments on all patients		
9. Identifies appropriate nursing interventions for alterations in level of consciousness		
B. With Direction, Provides Nursing Care to Patients with Impaired Mobility		
1. Knowledgeably administers reversal agents for neuromuscular blockade:		
a. Identifies neuromuscular blockade		

Postanesthesia Nursing Competencies *Continued* Level I/Step 1	Comments/Goals	Competency Met Date and Initial
b. Identifies signs of reversal		
c. Identifies two common neuromuscular blocking agents and anticipates their duration of effect		
d. Administers the common neuromuscular blocking reversal agent correctly		
2. Monitors recovery from neuromuscular blockade		
3. Identifies patients who have had regional anesthesia		
4. Initiates assessment of dermatome levels		
5. Identifies appropriate nursing interventions and considerations for patients with impaired mobility:		

Continued on following page

Postanesthesia Nursing Competencies *Continued* Level I/Step 1	Comments/Goals	Competency Met Date and Initial
a. Assesses extent of movement and sensation		
b. Assesses for and prevents injury to limbs and skin		
c. Assesses for distended bladder		
d. Documents agents used and any anesthetic complications		
IV. Participates in Professional Growth and Development		
A. Takes Initiative in Own Professional Growth		
1. Recognizes areas of personal strengths and weakness		
2. Reviews clinical work with senior nurse		

Continued on following page

Postanesthesia Nursing Competencies *Continued* Level I/Step 1	Comments/Goals	Competency Met Date and Initial
3. Follows through with suggestions for improvement in own clinical performance		
4. Assists with admissions and vital signs on patients other than her/his own		
5. Follows through with delegated work		
6. Attends staff meetings		

_____ has achieved Level I/Step 1 Beginner Postanesthesia Nursing proficiency.

_____   _____

Manager   Date

Level I/Step 2

I. Provides Nursing Care to Patients with Alterations in Health Management
   A. Demonstrates competency in caring for stable, complex patients and extended-care patients
   B. Manages the care of multiple patients
   C. Provides for the psychosocial support of the patient
   D. Provides for continuity of care
II. Provides Nursing Care to Patients with Alterations in Activity-Exercise Patterns
   A. With minimal supervision, provides nursing care for patients with potential for respiratory dysfunction
   B. With minimal supervision, provides nursing care for patients with potential for alterations in cardiac output
III. Provides Nursing Care to Patients with Alterations in Cognitive and Perceptual Patterns
   A. With minimal supervision, provides nursing care to patients with alterations in level of consciousness
   B. With minimal supervision, provides nursing care to patients with impaired mobility
IV. Participates in Professional Growth and Development
   A. Assumes responsibility for quality of care rendered

Postanesthesia Nursing Knowledge Level I/Step 2	Comments/Goals	Competency Met Date and Initial
I. Provides Nursing Care to Patients with Alterations in Health Management		
1. Lists responsibilities carried out for all extended-care and critical-care patients on all three shifts		
2. Discusses their implementation of the 13 commonly used nursing diagnoses for postanesthesia patients		
3. Locates proper reference material for laboratory results and lists norms for blood work		
4. Locates equipment manuals		
5. Lists signs and symptoms of the various blood reactions and describes nursing intervention		
6. Describes several methods, other than medications, for relieving pain and anxiety		
7. Describes preoperative teaching concepts as explained in the PACU self-instructional		
8. States the rationale for patient care conferences		

Continued on following page

Postanesthesia Nursing Knowledge *Continued* Level I/Step 2	Comments/Goals	Competency Met Date and Initial
II. Provides Nursing Care to Patients with Alterations in Activity-Exercise Patterns		
1. Discusses the importance of various types of breath sounds		
2. Describes the symptoms of an improperly placed endotracheal tube		
3. Explains the rationale for oxygen therapy in the immediate postanesthesia period		
4. Differentiates between low-flow and high-flow oxygen devices		
5. Differentiates between the PM 2 ambu bag and the Aires-T (black anesthesia) ventilatory bag		
6. Describes nursing responsibilities of the patient on a volume ventilator		
7. Defines CPAP and PEEP		

Continued on following page

Postanesthesia Nursing Knowledge *Continued* Level I/Step 2	Comments/Goals	Competency Met Date and Initial
8. Lists actions, dosage, and common side effect of emergency drugs:		
a. Sodium bicarbonate		
b. Epinephrine		
c. Calcium chloride		
d. Adenosine		
e. Procainamide		
f. Bretylium		

Continued on following page

Postanesthesia Nursing Knowledge *Continued* Level I/Step 2	Comments/Goals	Competency Met Date and Initial
9. Describes factors that contribute to hypotension and hypertension		
10. Lists actions, dosage parameters, and side effects of nitropruside and nitroglycerin		
11. Calculates dosages and rates for vasoactive drugs		
12. Descibes the cardiac conduction system		
13. Differentiates between the three heart block rhythms		
14. Describes pacemaker spikes		
15. Describes the Allen test and lists the complications of arterial catheterization		

Continued on following page

Postanesthesia Nursing Knowledge *Continued* Level I/Step 2	Comments/Goals	Competency Met Date and Initial
16. States nursing responsibilities for pulmonary artery catheter, and locates the PACU Hemodynamic Monitoring Manual		
17. Discusses nursing interventions that correspond to possible complications to patients with pulmonary artery catheters		
18. Describes equipment set-up, paddle placement, and energy dose for ventricular defibrillation		

Postanesthesia Nursing Knowledge *Continued* Level I/Step 2	Comments/Goals	Competency Met Date and Initial
III. Provides Nursing Care to Patients with Alterations in Cognitive and Perceptual Patterns		
1. Defines balanced anesthesia		
2. Lists interactions between anesthesia agents and perioperative medications		
3. Discusses reasons for the reversal or non-reversal of patients who have received narcotics and sedatives		
4. Describes four different inhalation agents, their emergence time, and primary side effect		
5. Describes the major symptoms that are associated with each of the stages of anesthesia		
6. Discusses nursing interventions to prevent emergence delirium		
7. Describes action, normal doses, and expected length of recovery for one depolarizing agent and three nondepolarizing agents		

Continued on following page

Postanesthesia Nursing Knowledge *Continued* Level I/Step 2	Comments/Goals	Competency Met Date and Initial
8. Discusses reasons for reversal or nonreversal of patients who have received neuromuscular blocking agents		
9. Lists the signs of recurarization		
10. Describes four frequently used regional anesthetic agents, including usual dose, expected recovery time, and two side effects		
11. Describes the effects of the vasopressor drug that is frequently used with regional anesthetics		

Postanesthesia Nursing Competencies Level I/Step 2	Comments/Goals	Competency Met Date and Initial
I. Provides Nursing Care to Patients with Alterations in Health Care Management		
A. Demonstrates Competency in Caring for Stable, Complex Patients and Extended-Care Patients		
1. Follows through on responsibilities for extended-care patients and critical-care patients		
2. Implements the plan of care for extended-care patients and complex patients		
3. Recognizes norms for all blood work		
4. Consistently and independently notifies appropriate physicians of laboratory results, x-rays and EKGs		
5. Troubleshoots monitors and bedside equipment		
6. Recognizes signs and symptoms of blood reactions		
7. Initiates nursing interventions when blood reactions occur		

Continued on following page

Postanesthesia Nursing Competencies *Continued* Level I/Step 2	Comments/Goals	Competency Met Date and Initial
8. Recognizes overt signs of patient deterioration; consults with senior or charge nurse and implements nursing interventions		
9. Identifies patients in need of steroid therapy		
B. Manages the Care of Multiple Patients		
1. Completes all admission assessments in a timely manner		
2. Initiates, follows through with, and evaluates the plan of care for noncomplex and complex, stable patients		
3. Implements the plan of care with supervision for complex, unstable patients		
4. Judges relative importance of different aspects of patient situations and prioritizes care for own caseload		
5. Discharges patients in an efficient and timely manner		

Continued on following page

Postanesthesia Nursing Competencies *Continued* Level I/Step 2	Comments/Goals	Competency Met Date and Initial
C. Provides for Psychosocial Support of the Patient		
1. Recognizes psychological distress related to post-operative pain, anxiety, or fear		
2. Initiates measure to relieve distress		
3. Responds to a therapeutic manner to patient's behaviors		
4. Allows for family visitation		
5. Preoperatively teaches, utilizing the PACU guidelines		
D. Provides for Continuity of Care		
1. Identifies and documents nursing diagnoses and interventions		
2. Utilizes appropriate terms for nursing plans of care		
3. Consults pertinent others for health data (i.e., medical services, nursing services, family)		

Continued on following page

Postanesthesia Nursing Competencies *Continued* Level I/Step 2	Comments/Goals	Competency Met Date and Initial
4. Gives accurate, concise, and organized patient reports		
II. Provides Nursing Care to Patients with Alterations in Activity-Exercise Patterns		
A. With Minimal Supervision, Provides Care to Patients with Potential for Respiratory Dysfunction		
1. Identifies rationale for oxygen therapy in various postanesthesia situations		
2. Independently initiates oxygen therapy to patients experiencing respiratory distress		
3. Describes characteristics of various breath sounds and relates them to patient care considerations		
4. Effectively ventilates with ambu bag and mask		
5. Prepares for endotracheal intubation		
6. Recognizes endotracheal tube displacement and refers situation immediately to appropriate person		
7. Independently regulates ventilator		

Postanesthesia Nursing Competencies *Continued* Level I/Step 2	Comments/Goals	Competency Met Date and Initial
8. Differentiates between pressure-sensitive and volume-regulated ventilators		
9. Monitors patient response to the ventilator		
10. Manages respiratory distress calmly and promptly		
11. Locates the CPAP equipment		
B. With Minimal Supervision, Provides Nursing Care to Patients with Potential for Alterations in Cardiac Output		
1. Knowledgeably administers emergency drugs:		
a. Locates emergency drug box		
b. Explains major use and usual dose for sodium bicarbonate, epinephrine, calcium chloride, and bretylium		

Continued on following page

Postanesthesia Nursing Competencies *Continued* Level I/Step 2	Comments/Goals	Competency Met Date and Initial
2. Initiates warming techniques		
3. Independently administers blood products according to protocols		
4. Calculates heart rate from rhythm strip		
5. Identifies P, QRS, T waves and measures PR and QRS intervals		
6. Traces cardiac conduction system through the heart		
7. Identifies heart blocks		
8. Identifies pacer spikes		

Continued on following page

Postanesthesia Nursing Competencies *Continued* Level I/Step 2	Comments/Goals	Competency Met Date and Initial
9. Initiates nursing measures to troubleshoot abnormal arterial waveforms		
10. Recognizes complications of arterial cannulation		
11. Identifies patient factors that contribute to hypotension and hypertension		
12. Compares reasons for using nitroprusside versus nitroglycerin		
13. Knowledgeably titrates vasoactive drugs		
14. Identifies normal pulmonary artery catheter waveforms		
15. Initiates nursing care for patients with pulmonary artery catheters		
16. Demonstrates correct set-up for and defibrillation of patients in ventricular fibrillation		

Continued on following page

Postanesthesia Nursing Competencies *Continued* Level I/Step 2	Comments/Goals	Competency Met Date and Initial
III. Provides Nursing Care to Patients with Alterations in Cognitive and Perceptual Patterns		
A. With Minimal Supervision, Provides Nursing Care to Patients with Alterations in Level of Consciousness		
1. Differentiates between balanced and neuroleptic anesthesia		
2. Recognizes symptoms of potentiation between anesthesia agents		
3. Recognizes indication of reversal or nonreversal of patients who have received narcotics or sedatives		
4. Recognizes side effects and anticipates emergency time for four different inhalation anesthetic agents		
5. Recognizes the major symptoms that are associated with each of the stages of anesthesia		
6. Identifies which stage of anesthesia the patient is in on admission and initiates appropriate nursing care		
7. Initiates nursing interventions when a patient is experiencing emergence delirium		

Continued on following page

Postanesthesia Nursing Competencies *Continued* Level I/Step 2	Comments/Goals	Competency Met Date and Initial
8. Predicts the length of expected recovery from anesthesia		
B. With Minimal Supervision, Provides Care to Patients with Impaired Mobility		
1. Differentiates between depolarizing and nondepolarizing neuromuscular blocking		
2. Anticipates when different neuromuscular blocking agents would be used		
3. Anticipates expected length of recovery from the neuromuscular agent used		
4. Predicts when reversal or nonreversal of the neuromuscular blockade would be beneficial to the patient		
5. Recognizes recurarization and promptly initiates nursing intervention		
6. Differentiates between types of regional anesthesia techniques (i.e., axillary block, Bier block, spinal, epidural, etc.)		

Continued on following page

Postanesthesia Nursing Competencies *Continued* Level I/Step 2	Comments/Goals	Competency Met Date and Initial
7. Recognizes potential problems related to regional anesthesia		
8. Predicts the length of recovery from regional anesthetics		
9. Plans, implements and evaluates nursing interventions for all patients having had regional anesthesia		
10. Promptly discharges patients after they achieve the discharge criteria for regional anesthesia		
IV. Participates in Professional Development and Growth		
A. Assumes Responsibility for Quality of Care Rendered		
1. Effectively organizes priorities of care for own patients		
2. Collaborates with senior nurses on clinical judgments and decisions		

Continued on following page

Postanesthesia Nursing Competencies *Continued* Level I/Step 2	Comments/Goals	Competency Met Date and Initial
3. Evaluates own nursing diagnoses for effectiveness		
4. Recognizes co-workers' needs and assists them consistently		
5. Seeks out work to be done		
6. Participates in staff meeting discussions		
7. Participates in patient care conference		
8. Evaluates own accomplishments and sets goals for oneself		

_____ has achieved Level I/Step 2 Beginner Postanesthesia Nursing proficiency.

_____   _____

Manager   Date

3

Post Anesthesia Nurse

Level II

I. Provides Nursing Care to Patients with Alterations in Health Management
   A. Demonstrates competency in caring for unstable, complex patients
   B. Provides for the coordination of patient care activities

II. Provides Nursing Care to Patients with Alterations in Activity-Exercise Patterns
   A. Independently provides nursing care to patients with complex respiratory dysfunction
   B. Independently provides nursing care to patients with complex alterations in cardiac output

III. Provides Nursing Care to Patients with Alterations in Cognitive and Perceptual Patterns
   A. Independently provides nursing care to patients with alterations in level of consciousness
   B. Independently provides nursing care to patients with impaired mobility

IV. Participates in Professional Growth and Development
   A. Provides for clinical supervision
   B. Takes initiative to identify quality improvement issues

Postanesthesia Nursing Knowledge Level II	Comments/Goals	Competency Met Date and Initial
I. Provides Nursing Care to Patients with Alterations in Health Management		
1. Describes how they implement the nursing process in their daily nursing care		
2. Identifies legal aspects of proper documentation		
3. Discusses one element related to legalities of their own documentation		
4. Describes malignant hyperthermia and lists nursing implications		
II. Provides Nursing Care to Patients with Alterations in Activity—Exercise Patterns		
1. Defines common factors that contribute to airway obstruction		
2. Lists common factors that contribute to hypoxia and hypercarbia		
3. Explains ways to prevent and treat hypoxia and hypercarbia		
4. Analyzes components of arterial blood gases		

Continued on following page

Postanesthesia Nursing Knowledge *Continued* Level II	Comments/Goals	Competency Met Date and Initial
5. Explains differences in oxygen therapy for patients with COPD		
6. Explains pressure support ventilation		
7. Describes pediatric airway anatomy and discusses the signs of pediatric respiratory distress		
8. Explains nursing implications for pediatric airway management		
9. Lists common bronchodilator agents used in the PACU, describing usual dosage and side effect of each		
10. Discusses respiratory physiology as it pertains to CPAP and PEEP		
11. Discusses chest x-ray findings in relation to nursing care		

Continued on following page

Postanesthesia Nursing Knowledge *Continued* Level II	Comments/Goals	Competency Met Date and Initial
12. Lists the actions, dosage, and one side effect of glycopyrrolate (Robinol)		
13. Discusses factors that effect myocardial workload, defining preload, afterload, and Starling's law		
14. Lists actions, dosage, and two side effects of dopamine and dobutamine		
15. Lists actions, dosage, and two side effects of beta blockers and calcium channel blockers		

III. Provides Nursing Care to Patients with Alterations in Cognitive and Perceptual Patterns

1. Explains the concepts of solubility and distribution of agents in relation to emergence time		
2. Discusses the thermal effects on emergence time		
3. Discusses own patient experiences of delayed emergence, relating the patient factors that contributed to it		

Continued on following page

Postanesthesia Nursing Knowledge *Continued* Level II	Comments/Goals	Competency Met Date and Initial
4. Describes four situations in which physostigmine (Antilirium) could be used as a reversal agent		
5. Discusses the causes and complications of shivering; lists nursing implications		
6. Compares the advantages and disadvantages of four major nondepolarizing agents (tubocurarine, pancuronium, metacurine, atracurium)		
7. Compares the advantages and disadvantages of the three reversal agents (neostigmine, pyridostigmine, edrophonium)		
8. Describes why some antibiotics tend to interact with neuromuscular blocking agents		

Postanesssthesia Nursing Knowledge *Continued* Level II	Comments/Goals	Competency Met Date and Initial
IV. Participates in Professional Growth and Development		
1. Describes nurse coordinator responsibilities		
2. Identifies resources and proper channels of communication for problem solving the unit management problems		
3. Discusses ways to uphold the PACU standards of care		
4. Describes the use of anecdotals in maintaining the standards of care		
5. Describes components of feedback and counseling		
6. Describes the goal-setting process		
7. Discusses proper documentation of unit management problems		

Continued on following page

Postanesthesia Nursing Competencies Level II	Comments/Goals	Competency Met Date and Initial
I. Provides Nursing Care to Patients with Alterations in Health Management		
A. Demonstrates Competency in Caring for Unstable, Complex Patients		
1. Identifies interrelated patient problems		
2. Anticipates potential patient crises, and initiates interventions to prevent them		
3. Implements effective nursing interventions when patient deterioration occurs		
4. Performs complicated nursing procedures		
5. Functions calmly and promptly in emergency situations		
6. Identifies symptoms of malignant hyperthermia		

Continued on following page

Postanesthesia Nursing Competencies *Continued* Level II	Comments/Goals	Competency Met Date and Initial
B. Provides for the Coordination of Patient Care Activities		
1. Identifies, implements, and evaluates the plan of care for all types of postanesthesia patients (non-complex, extended-care, complex, and unstable complex)		
2. Recognizes the health care team as an integral part of the effectiveness of patient care		
3. Identifies the needs of patients other than own case load; coordinates own patient care with co-worker's needs		
4. Actively cooperates with all health care team members to plan and coordinate care for the entire unit		
5. Maintains accurate documentation on all records		

Postanesthesia Nursing Competencies *Continued* Level II	Comments/Goals	Competency Met Date and Initial
II. Provides Nursing Care to Patients with Alterations in Activity-Exercise Patterns		
A. Independently Provides Nursing Care to Patients with Complex Respiratory Dysfunction		
1. Knowledgeably initiates and evaluates alternative oxygen therapy:		
a. Croup tent		
b. Venturi mask		
c. Non-rebreather mask		
2. Evaluates patient factors that contribute to hypoxia and hypercarbia		
3. Implements nursing measures to correct hypoxia and/or hypercarbia		
4. Analyzes and monitors results of arterial blood gas determinations		

Continued on following page

Postanesthesia Nursing Competencies *Continued* Level II	Comments/Goals	Competency Met Date and Initial
5. Initiates respiratory care for pediatric patients		
6. Appropriately positions and ventilates the pediatric patient		
7. Effectively ventilates with an Aires-T ventilatory bag (anesthesia black bag)		
8. Knowledgeably administers bronchodilator agents		
9. Administers aerosol treatments		
10. Troubleshoots the ventilator		
11. Identifies nursing implications related to chest x-ray findings		

Continued on following page

Postanesthesia Nursing Competencies *Continued* Level II	Comments/Goals	Competency Met Date and Initial
12. Effectively manages and evaluates the care of the patient with CPAP and PEEP		
B. Independently Provides Nursing Care to Patients with Complex Alterations in Cardiac Output		
1. Identifies patient factors that affect myocardial workload		
2. Identifies relationships between preload, afterload, and Starling's law and changes in the patient's blood pressure, pulmonary pressure, and cardiac output		
3. Compares the use of dopamine to that of dobutamine		
4. Compares the use of beta blockers to that of calcium channel blockers		
5. Differentiates between atropine and glycopyrrolate		
6. Anticipates medical interventions and initiates nursing interventions to prevent and treat complications of the cardiovascular system (hemodynamic changes)		

Postanesthesia Nursing Competencies *Continued* Level II	Comments/Goals	Competency Met Date and Initial
III. Provides Nursing Care to Patients with Alterations in Cognitive and Perceptual Patterns		
A. Independently Provides Nursing Care to Patients with Alterations in Level of Consciousness		
1. Offers rationale for deviations from the normal recovery process:		
a. Relates the solubility and distribution factors		
b. Relates the potentiating drugs		
c. Relates thermal effects		
2. Knowledgeably administers physostigmine in four different patient situations		
3. Initiates treatment for postanesthesia shivering		
B. Independently Provides Nursing Care to Patients with Impaired Mobility		
1. Identifies one or two patient factors that contribute to the decision for the nondepolarizing agent chosen and the reversal agent chosen		
2. Recognizes the antibiotics that interact with muscle relaxants		

Continued on following page

Postanesthesia Nursing Competencies *Continued* Level II	Comments/Goals	Competency Met Date and Initial
IV. Participates in Professional Growth and Development		
A. Provides for Clinical Supervision		
1. Takes charge of the unit for one shift with general supervision:		
a. Handles desk work effectively		
b. Coordinates patient care assignments		
c. Delegates work to be done		
2. Utilizes appropriate problem-solving techniques		
3. Identifies the standard of care rendered		
4. Assists in the responsibilities of upholding the PACU standards of care		

Continued on following page

Postanesthesia Nursing Competencies *Continued* Level II	Comments/Goals	Competency Met Date and Initial
B. Takes Initiative to Identify Quality Improvement Problems		
1. Identifies unsafe patient care practice or deviations from the standards of care		
2. Communicates and documents problems to shift manager		
3. Offers constructive suggestions for problem management		

_____ has achieved Level II Postanesthesia Nursing proficiency.

_____   _____

Manager   Date

4

Senior Post Anesthesia Nurse

Level III

I. Provides Nursing Care to Patients with Alterations in Health Management
   A. Demonstrates competency in caring for the whole patient rather than aspects of patient care
   B. Maintains accountability for own nursing judgments and actions
II. Provides Nursing Care to Patients with Alterations in Activity-Exercise Patterns
   A. Provides alternatives in the care of patients with complex respiratory dysfunction
   B. Provides alternatives in the care of patients with complex alterations in cardiac output
III. Provides Nursing Care to Patients with Alterations in Cognitive and Perceptual Patterns
   A. Provides alternatives in the care of patients with complex alterations in level of consciousness
   B. Provides alternatives in the care of patients with extended impairment of mobility
IV. Participates in Professional Growth and Development
   A. Provides for and acts as a resource for clinical supervision
   B. Participates in clinical education activities
   C. Participates in quality improvement activities

Postanesthesia Nursing Knowledge Level III	Comments/Goals	Competency Met Date and Initial
I. Provides Nursing Care to Patients with Alterations in Health Management		
1. Expands their knowledge in regards to the inter-related reactions of all body systems in response to the anesthetic process		
2. Discusses qualitative distinctions in patient status		
3. Formulates alternatives for patient care management		
4. Analyzes physiologic responses in relation to peri-operative stress		
5. Discusses methods of incorporating the patient and family in the postanesthesia care plan		
6. Discusses the anesthetic course specific to pediatrics and makes distinctions in plans for care for pediatric patients		
7. Describes one or two situations where nursing care had a substantial impact on the progress of the patient's recovery		

Continued on following page

Postanesthesia Nursing Knowledge *Continued* Level III	Comments/Goals	Competency Met Date and Initial
II. Provides Nursing Care to Patients with Alterations in Activity-Exercise Patterns		
1. Differentiates between the various types of shock, defines medical treatment, and describes nursing care management		
2. Compares cardioversion to defibrillation		
3. Describes different types of pacemakers and discusses proper functioning of pacemakers		
4. Expands knowledge of the pulmonary artery catheter and patient care management		

Continued on following page

Postanesthesia Nursing Knowledge *Continued* Level III	Comments/Goals	Competency Met Date and Initial
III. Provides Nursing Care to Patients with Alterations in Cognitive and Perceptual Patterns		
1. Evaluates new anesthetic agents, identifying complications and formulating nursing care plans according to nursing implications		
2. Explains the concept of minimum alveolar concentration (MAC) in relation to the level of anesthesia		
3. Relates how these factors influence the effects of neuromuscular blocking agents:		
a. Fluid balance		
b. Na^+, K^+, Ca^+, Mg^+		
c. pH, CO_2		
d. Epinephrine, norepinephrine		
e. Lidocaine, quinidine		

Postanesthesia Nursing Knowledge *Continued* Level III	Comments/Goals	Competency Met Date and Initial
f. Narcotics, sedatives		
IV. Participates in Professional Growth and Development		
1. Describes leadership qualities		
2. Discusses the roles delegation and collaboration play in day-to-day unit management		
3. Describes the role research findings play in their present nursing care		
4. Discusses proper modes of initiating change in the unit		
5. Evaluates the value of setting goals		
6. Discusses alternatives for self-improvement		

Continued on following page

Postanesthesia Nursing Competency Level III	Comments/Goals	Competency Met Date and Initial
I. Provides Nursing Care to Patients with Alterations in Health Management		
A. Demonstrates Competency in Caring for the Patient as a Whole Rather than Aspects of Patient Care		
1. Identifies and relates knowledge of neurological, vascular, renal, and cardiopulmonary systems to postanesthesia care		
2. Evaluates physiological responses in relation to the stress of the operative period		
3. Judges qualitative distinctions in patient presentations and initiates care based on these distinctions (perceptual knowledge)		
4. Provides alternatives to patients in multisystem crises		
5. Effectively manages the complex pediatric patient		
6. Effectively manages the care of the patient who sustains malignant hyperthermia		
7. Applies experience and knowledge of expected outcomes to the plans of care and incorporates long-term goals		

Continued on following page

Postanesthesia Nursing Competency *Continued* Level III	Comments/Goals	Competency Met Date and Initial
8. Provides patient with opportunities to participate in plan of care		
9. Adapts to patient's level and pace of development, respecting patient's interpretation of illness		
10. Alters plan of care as a result of covert or subtle patient cues (i.e., recognizes patient problems prior to explicit changes in vital signs or status)		
11. Uses discretionary judgment (i.e., weighs the need for rest and comfort versus the therapeutic regimen)		
B. Maintains Accountability for Own Nursing Judgments and Actions		

Continued on following page

Postanesthesia Nursing Competency *Continued* Level III	Comments/Goals	Competency Met Date and Initial
II. Provides Nursing Care to Patients with Alterations in Activity-Exercise Patterns		
A. Provides Alternatives to Patients with Complex Respiratory Dysfunction		
B. Provides Alternatives to Patients with Complex Alterations in Cardiac Output		
1. Clinically identifies the signs for the various types of shock		
2. Anticipates medical interventions and initiates nursing interventions for the various types of shock		
3. Identifies malfunctioning pacemakers		
4. Anticipates and sets up for cardioversion		
5. Troubleshoots the pulmonary artery catheter monitoring system		
6. Relates pulmonary pressures and cardiac output measurements to patient status and predicted outcomes		

Continued on following page

Postanesthesia Nursing Competencies *Continued* Level III	Comments/Goals	Competency Met Date and Initial
III. Provides Nursing Care to Patients with Alterations in Cognitive and Perceptual Patterns		
A. Provides Alternatives in the Care of Patients with Complex Alterations in Level of Consciousness		
1. Identifies new anesthesia agents, their complications, and implications for postanesthesia care		
2. Relates the concept of MAC to the level of consciousness on admission and the progression of recovery		
3. Identifies the clinical course and initiates nursing interventions to the anesthetic course specific to pediatrics		
B. Provides Alternatives in the Care of Patients with Extended Impairment of Mobility		
1. Anticipates clinical effects of these factors in relation to neuromuscular blocking agents:		
a. Fluid balance		
b. Electrolyte balance		
c. Arterial blood gases		

Continued on following page

Postanesthesia Nursing Competency Level III	Comments/Goals	Competency Met Date and Initial
d. Catecholamines		
e. Depressant agents		
2. Identifies dual block		
3. Effectively manages the patient who has sustained an extended impairment of mobility (from muscle relaxants or regional anesthetics)		

Continued on following page

Postanesthesia Nursing Competencies *Continued* Level III	Comments/Goals	Competency Met Date and Initial
IV. Participates in Professional Growth and Development		
A. Provides for and Acts as a Resource for Clinical Supervision		
1. Effectively manages and coordinates nursing staff for a specific shift:		
a. Takes a leadership role in directing personnel		
b. Identifies day-to-day problems		
c. Institutes corrective measures for day-to-day problems		
d. Makes independent decisions		
e. Holds others accountable for their behavior and decisions		
f. Assumes charge role in emergency situations, needing minimal resources from co-workers		

Continued on following page

Postanesthesia Nursing Competency *Continued* Level III	Comments/Goals	Competency Met Date and Initial
2. Monitors and maintains nursing standards of care as primary care-giver or coordinator nurse		
3. Assist with the evaluation of co-workers:		
a. Initiates bedside feedback and counseling		
b. Consistently writes anecdotals		
B. Participates in Clinical Education Activities		
1. Updates own knowledge through inquiry and independent study		
2. Teaches staff utilizing past and present clinical experience		
3. Assists others in evaluating the effectiveness of nursing care rendered		

Continued on following page

Postanesthesia Nursing Competency *Continued* Level III	Comments/Goals	Competency Met Date and Initial
4. Proposes alternatives for self-improvement		
C. Participates in Quality Improvement Activities		
1. Offers positive suggestions for identified problems and/or researchable problems		
2. Cooperates and follows through with research activities and/or planned change		

_____ has achieved Level III Senior Postanesthesia Nursing proficiency.

_____
Manager

_____
Date

5

Advanced Post Anesthesia Nurse

Level IV/Step 1

I. Provides Nursing Care to Patients with Alterations in Health Management
    A. Demonstrates autonomy in rendering care and clinical decision-making
    B. Demonstrates competency in managing multiproblem nursing situations
II. Participates in Professional Growth and Development
    A. Monitors and maintains a therapeutic environment for staff and patients
    B. Acts as catalyst for change in the grooming process
    C. Participates in clinical education activities

Postanesthesia Nursing Knowledge Level IV/Step 1	Comments/Goals	Competency Met Date and Initial
I. Provides Nursing Care to Patients with Alterations in Health Management		
1. Formulates and describes their leadership style		
2. Discusses what risk-taking means to them		
3. Describes patient care situation that indicates high-level clinical decision-making capabilities		
4. Analyzes and evaluates researchable data in relation to postanesthesia nursing care		
5. Compares CCF's postanesthesia nursing practice to that of other hospitals		

Continued on following page

Postanesthesia Nursing Knowledge *Continued* Level IV/Step 1	Comments/Goals	Competency Met Date and Initial
II. Participates in Professional Growth and Development		
1. Discusses what a therapeutic recovery unit environment means to them		
2. Proposes ways to maintain an atmosphere of open communication and trust		
3. Develops and describes own method of feedback and counseling		
4. Describes methods of conflict resolution		
5. Evaluates alternatives in peer grooming process		
6. Differentiates between androgogical and pedagogical teaching methods		
7. Discusses alternatives for teaching and learning		
8. Describes the preceptor role, indicating its value in the PACU		

Continued on following page

Postanesthesia Nursing Competencies Level IV/Step 1	Comments/Goals	Competency Met Date and Initial
I. Provides Nursing Care to Patients with Alterations in Health Management		
A. Demonstrates Autonomy in Rendering Care and Clinical Decision-Making		
1. Makes independent judgments and initiates follow-through; seeks consultation appropriately		
2. Applies current nursing research findings to clinical practice		
3. Evaluates effectiveness of nursing care standards and nursing care rendered in relation to patient outcome		
4. Adjusts nursing care and clinical decisions based on predicted and observed patient outcome		
B. Demonstrates Competency in Managing Multi-Problem Nursing Situations		
1. Judges qualitative situations involving multiple variables		
2. "Hones in" on accurate region of preventing problems		
3. Predicts outcomes based on knowledge and clinical experience		

Continued on following page

Postanesthesia Nursing Competencies *Continued* Level IV/Step 1	Comments/Goals	Competency Met Date and Initial
4. Effectively manages routine standards, procedures, and guidelines in the context of multiple care needs		

II. Participates in Professional Growth and Development

A. Monitors and Maintains a Therapeutic Environment for Staff and Patients

1. Anticipates potential problems and manages staff accordingly		
2. Plans for next shift staffing needs, anticipating staffing needs for the next 24 hours		
3. Utilizes resources within the milieu to provide for problem-solving		
4. Creates an atmosphere of trust, confidence, and open communication		
5. Uses discretionary judgment in patient care assignments (correlates nursing skill level with patient activity)		
6. Independently takes charge role or acts as a resource in emergency situations		

Continued on following page

Postanesthesia Nursing Competencies Level IV/Step 1	Comments/Goals	Competency Met Date and Initial
B. Acts as Catalyst for Change in the Grooming Process		
1. Initiates counseling on complex issues and communicates same to managers		
2. Write informative and ongoing anecdotal notes		
3. Follows through after counseling, as guided by manager		
C. Participates in Clinical Education Activities		
1. Updates own knowledge through self-motivated independent study; goes after learning experiences		
2. Assists others in evaluation of nursing care standards, nursing care rendered, and patient outcomes		
3. Shares information from various resources and current research for maintaining quality nursing care in a formal manner		
4. Participates in exploring nursing issues related to clinical practice		

Continued on following page

Postanesthesia Nursing Competencies Level IV/Step 1	Comments/Goals	Competency Met Date and Initial
5. Collaborates with health care team members in evaluating and implementing planned change		
6. Acts as preceptor for nursing personnel, implementing clinical instruction based on mutual goals.		

_____ has achieved Level IV/Step 1 Advanced Postanesthesia Nursing proficiency.

_____   _____

Manager   Date

LEVEL IV/STEP 2

I. Provides Nursing Care to Patients with Alterations in Health Management

    A. Effectively manages and coordinates complex and changing patient care needs and staffing needs

II. Participates in Professional Growth and Development

    A. Participates in activities that contribute to development of a professional body of knowledge with emphasis on the specialty of postanesthesia care

    B. Acts as change agent in the grooming process

Postanesthesia Nursing Competencies Level IV/Step 2	Comments/Goals	Competency Met Date and Initial
I. Provides Nursing Care to Patients with Alterations in Health Management		
A. Effectively Manages and Coordinates Complex and Changing Patient Care Needs and Staffing Needs		
1. Recognizes the needs of the entire unit at any given time and offers assistance, suggestions, and alternatives when needed		
2. Remains flexible within the organization of the unit, promptly recognizing changing needs, evaluating effectiveness of current plan, and promptly altering the plan as necessary		
3. Takes risks based on secure and accurate judgments, in both unit needs and patient care needs		
II. Participates in Professional Growth and Development		
A. Participates in Activities that Contribute to the Development of a Professional Body of Knowledge, with Emphasis on the Speciality of Postanesthesia Care		
B. Acts as Change Agent in the Grooming Process		
1. Creates an atmosphere that promotes evaluation of nursing care and nursing standards		
2. Takes a leadership role in assisting others to identify, evaluate, and maintain nursing standards of care		

Continued on following page

Postanesthesia Nursing Competencies *Continued* Level IV/Step 2	Comments/Goals	Competency Met Date and Initial
3. Assists others in exploring education opportunities to promote professional development		
4. Provides opportunities for other personnel to attain clinical knowledge and develop clinical skills		
5. Facilitates behavior modification on an individual basis		
6. Follows through with the process of behavior modification on a long-term basis		
7. Assists others in goal-setting		
8. Participates in peer evaluation		

_____ has achieved Level IV/Step 2 Advanced Postanesthesia Nursing proficiency.

_____   _____
Manager   Date

PART TWO

PREANESTHESIA NURSING KNOWLEDGE BASE AND CLINICAL COMPETENCIES

Definition of Preanesthesia Nursing

Preanesthesia nursing is an area of professional nursing practice that renders acute care by specially educated nursing personnel who have the ability to recognize and manage the problems particular to preanesthesia patients. Preanesthesia nurses specialize in meeting immediate preoperative teaching needs for both patient and family, recognizing and managing anxiety and fear, and coordinating preanesthesia/presurgical preparation

6

Beginner Pre Anesthesia Nurse

Level I

I. Provides Nursing Care to Patients with Alterations in Health Management

    A. With direction, demonstrates competency in caring for preanesthesia patients and their families or significant others

    B. Provides for communication of health data to interdepartmental professional services

II. Provides Nursing Care to Patients with Alterations in Activity-Exercise Patterns

    A. With minimal supervision, provides nursing care for patients with alterations in fluid volume (deficit)

    B. With minimal supervision, provides nursing care to patients with potential for physical injury

    C. With minimal supervision, provides nursing care for patients with potential for respiratory dysfunction

III. Provides Nursing Care to Patients with Alterations in Cognitive and Perceptual Patterns

    A. With minimal supervision, provides nursing care for patients with anxiety

    B. With minimal supervision, provides nursing care for patients with a knowledge deficit

    C. With minimal supervision, provides nursing care for patients with potential for noncompliance (denial of illness)

    D. With minimal supervision, provides nursing care for patients with ineffective coping skills

IV. Participates in Professional Growth and Development

    A. Assumes responsibility for quality of care rendered

    B. Takes initiative in own professional growth

Preanesthesia Nursing Knowledge Level I/Step 1	Comments/Goals	Competency Met Date and Initial
I. Provides Nursing Care to Patients with Alterations in Health Management		
1. Discusses their interpretation of the various aspects of preanesthesia nursing		
2. Lists responsibilities carried out for all preoperative patients		
3. Locates proper reference materials		
4. Discusses the requirements for patient admission		
5. Lists the components of the preoperative admission packet		
6. Discusses the importance and the components of the Preoperative Patient Education Record		
7. Discusses the requirements for patient discharge to the operating room		
8. Describes the role of the family and/or significant other(s) in the preoperative phase		

Continued on following page

Preanesthesia Nursing Knowledge *Continued* Level I/Step 1	Comments/Goals	Competency Met Date and Initial
9. Describes the roles and responsibilities of the staff, support staff, physicians, and other interdepartmental services		
10. Describes the role of the pediatric core group and differentiates between the childlife worker role in the preanesthesia phase		
11. Discusses the role of anesthesia clearance and PreCare (Holding area)		

Preanesthesia Nursing Knowledge Level I/Step 1	Comments/Goals	Competency Met Date and Initial
II. Provides Nursing Care to Patients with Alterations in Activity-Exercise Patterns		
1. Discusses the importance of patients being NPO prior to surgery; differentiates between adults and pediatric patients		
2. States the IV protocols for preoperative patients		
3. Discusses safety measures pertinent to preanesthesia care		
4. States who is responsible for preoperative medication orders (i.e., narcotics, sedatives)		
5. Discusses the dosage and correct administration of naloxone (Narcan); states one side effect		
6. States the nursing responsibilities in regards to PCA teaching		
7. Defines the guidelines for monitored anesthesia care (MAC), local, regional, and general anesthesia		

Continued on following page

Preanesthesia Nursing Knowledge *Continued* Level I/Step 1	Comments/Goals	Competency Met Date and Initial
8. Lists actions, dosage and common side effects of:		
a. Antibiotics (cephalexin [Keflex], penicillin, vancomycin)		
b. Steroids (dexamethasone [Decadron], hydrocortisone PO_4)		
c. Narcotics (meperidine [Demerol], MSO_4, codeine)		
d. Sedatives (diazepam [Valium], midazolam [Versed], lorazepam [Ativan], chloral hydrate, triazolam [Halcion])		
e. Hydroxyzine (Vistaril) and scopolamine		
f. Ranitidine (Zantac)		

Continued on following page

Preanesthesia Nursing Knowledge *Continued* Level I/Step 1	Comments/Goals	Competency Met Date and Initial
III. Provides Nursing Care to Patients with Alterations in Cognitive and Perceptual Patterns		
1. Recognizes psychological distress related to preoperative fear or anxiety		
2. Discusses the different anxiety levels in relation to effective preoperative teaching		
3. Lists reasons patients may exhibit a knowledge deficit preoperatively		
4. Recognizes reasons patients demonstrate a non-compliant behavior (denial of illness) preoperatively		
5. Explains reasons that patients demonstrate ineffective coping skills preoperatively		
6. States the importance of including family and/or significant other(s) in assessing support systems		

Continued on following page

Preanesthesia Nursing Knowledge *Continued* Level I/Step 1	Comments/Goals	Competency Met Date and Initial
IV. Participates in Professional Growth and Development		
1. Explains the importance of priorities		
2. Discusses communication and collaboration with senior nurses on clinical judgments and decisions		
3. Recognizes areas of personal strengths and weaknesses		
4. States the rationale for patient care conferences		

Continued on following page

Preanesthesia Nursing Competencies Level I/Step 2	Comments/Goals	Competency Met Date and Initial
I. Provides Nursing Care to Patients with Alterations in Health Management		
1. Follows through on all problems and responsibilities for preanesthesia patients		
2. Initiates the preoperative admission procedures:		
a. Includes preoperative checklist, preoperative questionnaire, patient education record, and valuables and belongings list		
b. Pediatric assessments		
c. Preoperative teaching		
d. Preoperative medications and other specific orders		
e. Notification to proper service of actual/potential problems		
f. Routines of different services (i.e., orthopedics, GYN, ENT, ophthalmology, etc.)		

Continued on following page

Preanesthesia Nursing Competencies *Continued* Level I/Step 2	Comments/Goals	Competency Met Date and Initial
g. Family and/or significant other(s)		
3. Completes admission assessments promptly using good priority-setting		
4. Implements appropriate plan of care and nursing interventions:		
a. Follows preanesthesia nursing guidelines, policies, and procedures		
b. Follows through with responsibilities for pre-anesthesia patients/families		
c. Includes family and/or significant other(s) in preoperative teaching		
5. Consistently notifies appropriate physicians and charge nurse of alterations in patient data		
6. Utilizes the proper reference material before implementing preoperative teaching for the various surgeries		

Continued on following page

Preanesthesia Nursing Competencies *Continued* Level I/Step 2	Comments/Goals	Competency Met Date and Initial
7. Knowledgeably administers preoperative medications (adult and pediatric):		
a. Antibiotics		
b. Steroids		
c. Narcotics		
d. Sedatives		
e. Hydroxyzine (Vistaril) and scopolamine		
f. Ranitidine (Zantac)		
8. Instructs patients/families on use of PCA pump		

Continued on following page

Preanesthesia Nursing Competencies *Continued* Level I/Step 2	Comments/Goals	Competency Met Date and Initial
9. Promptly discharges patients to the OR		
10. Performs the functions of the support staff		
11. Facilitates communication between the OR control desk, anesthesia control desk, OR personnel, anesthesia clearance and precare		
12. Communicates delays to patients/families		
13. Consistently communicates with the preanesthesia staff, support staff and PACU unit coordinator		

Continued on following page

Preanesthesia Nursing Competencies Level I/Step 2	Comments/Goals	Competency Met Date and Initial
II. Provides Nursing Care to Patients with Alterations in Activity-Exercise Patterns		
1. Identifies appropriate nursing interventions for patients who ate or drank after designated time		
2. Maintains side rails and crib rails in up position after administration of preoperative narcotic/sedative		
3. Assists patient to bathroom after a preoperative narcotic/sedative		
4. Intervenes appropriately for respiratory distress		

Continued on following page

Preanesthesia Nursing Competencies *Continued* Level I/Step 2	Comments/Goals	Competency Met Date and Initial
III. Provides Nursing Care to Patients with Alterations in Cognitive and Perceptual Patterns		
1. Initiates measures to relieve preoperative fears and anxiety		
2. Responds in a therapeutic manner to patient behaviors		
3. Preoperatively teaches according to patient's anxiety level		
4. Assesses the patient's level of knowledge with appropriate nursing interventions		
5. Assesses the patients' perception of illness and surgery with appropriate nursing interventions		
6. Assesses the patient's response to surgery with appropriate nursing interventions		
7. Allows for active family participation		

Continued on following page

Preanesthesia Nursing Competencies *Continued* Level I/Step 2	Comments/Goals	Competency Met Date and Initial
IV. Participates in Professional Growth and Development		
1. Effectively organizes priorities of care for own patients		
2. Collaborates with senior nurses on clinical judgments and decisions		
3. Recognizes co-workers' needs and assists them consistently		
4. Seeks out work to be done		
5. Participates in patient care conferences		

Continued on following page

Preanesthesia Nursing Competencies *Continued* Level I/Step 2	Comments/Goals	Competency Met Date and Initial
6. Participates in staff meeting discussions		
7. Evaluates own accomplishments and sets goals for oneself		

_____ has achieved Level I Beginner Preanesthesia Nursing proficiency.

_____   _____

Manager   Date

7

Pre Anesthesia Nurse

Level II

I. Provides Nursing Care to Patients with Alterations in Health Management
   A. Independently demonstrates competency in caring for complex preanesthesia patients and their families or significant others
   B. Provides for the coordination of patient care activities

II. Provides Nursing Care to Patients with Alterations in Activity-Exercise Patterns
   A. Independently provides nursing care for patients with alterations in fluid volume (deficit)
   B. Independently provides nursing care for patients with potential for physical injury
   C. Independently provides nursing care for patients with potential for respiratory dysfunction

III. Provides Nursing Care to Patients with Alterations in Cognitive and Perceptual Patterns
   A. Independently provides nursing care for patients with anxiety
   B. Independently provides nursing care for patients with a knowledge deficit
   C. Independently provides nursing care for patients with potential for noncompliance (denial of illness)

IV. Participates in Professional Growth and Development
   A. Provides for clinical supervision
   B. Takes initiative to identify quality improvement issues

Preanesthesia Nursing Competencies Level II	Comments/Goals	Competency Met Date and Initial
I. Provides Nursing Care to Patients with Alterations in Health Management		
1. Identifies interrelated preoperative patient problems		
2. Anticipates actual and potential preoperative patient problems and initiates appropriate interventions		
3. Recognizes the health care team as an integral part of the effectiveness of preanesthesia patient care		
4. Utilizes childlife worker as consultant for pediatric and adolescent patients		
5. Actively cooperates with all health care team members to plan and coordinate care for the entire unit		
6. Identifies the needs of the patients and families other than own case load		
7. Maintains accurate preoperative documentation on all records		

Continued on following page

Preanesthesia Nursing Competencies *Continued* Level II	Comments/Goals	Competency Met Date and Initial
II. Provides Nursing Care to Patients with Alterations in Activity-Exercise Patterns		
1. Knowledgeably initiates appropriate nursing interventions		
2. Takes leadership role in maintaining safety in the preanesthesia area		
3. Takes leadership role in emergency situations in the preanesthesia area		

Continued on following page

Preanesthesia Nursing Competencies *Continued* Level II	Comments/Goals	Competency Met Date and Initial
III. Provides Nursing Care to Patients with Alterations in Cognitive and Perceptual Patterns		
1. Offers rationale for deviations from the normal coping behavior mechanisms		
2. Initiates treatment for the patient and or significant other(s), utilizing appropriate referral services if necessary		

Continued on following page

Preanesthesia Nursing Competencies Continued Level II	Comments/Goals	Competency Met Date and Initial
IV. Participates in Professional Growth and Development		
1. Identifies unsafe preanesthesia patient care practice		
2. Takes charge of the unit for one shift:		
a. Identifies charge nurse responsibilities		
b. Takes a leadership role in directing personnel		
c. Makes independent decisions		
d. Anticipates potential problems and manages staff accordingly		
e. Holds others accountable for their behavior and decisions		
f. Handles desk work effectively		

Continued on following page

Preanesthesia Nursing Competencies *Continued* Level II	Comments/Goals	Competency Met Date and Initial
g. Coordinates patient flow within the preanesthesia area		
3. Utilizes resources and proper channels of communication in solving unit management problems		
4. Communicates and documents problems to shift manager		
5. Provides guidance to students and Level I nurses		
6. Offers constructive suggestions for identified problems		
7. Assists with the evaluation of co-workers:		
a. Initiates bedside feedback and counseling		
b. Follows through after counseling		

Continued on following page

Preanesthesia Nursing Competencies *Continued* Level II	Comments/Goals	Competency Met Date and Initial
8. Cooperates and follows through with researchable activities and/or planned changes		
9. Acts as preceptor for nursing personnel, implementing clinical instruction based on mutual goals		

_____ has achieved Level II Preanesthesia Nursing proficiency

_____   _____
Manager   Date

8

Senior Pre Anesthesia Nurse

Level III

I. Provides Nursing Care to Patients with Alterations in Health Management
   A. Demonstrates competency in caring for complex preanesthesia patients and their families or significant others
   B. Maintains accountability for own nursing judgments and actions
II. Participates in Professional Growth and Development
   A. Assumes responsibility for quality of care rendered
   B. Participates in clinical education activities
   C. Participates in quality improvement activities

Preanesthesia Nursing Competency Level III	Comments/Goals	Competency Met Date and Initial
I. Provides Nursing Care to Patients with Alterations in Health Management		
A. Demonstrates Competency in Caring for Complex Preanesthesia Patients and Their Families or Significant Others		
1. Effectively manages complex preanesthesia adult and pediatric patients as the "clinical expert"		
2. Alters plan of care as a result of covert or subtle patient cues (i.e., recognizes patient's problems as a result of preoperative teaching and following through)		
B. Maintains Accountability for Own Nursing Judgments and Actions		

Continued on following page

Preanesthesia Nursing Competency *Continued* Level III	Comments/Goals	Competency Met Date and Initial
II. Participates in Professional Growth and Development		
A. Assumes Responsibility for Quality of Care Rendered		
1. Monitors and maintains preanesthesia nursing standards of care as primary care-giver or coordinator nurse		
2. Assists with the evaluation of co-workers:		
a. Initiatives bedside feedback and teaching		
b. Consistently writes anecdotals		
B. Participates in Clinical Education Activities		
1. Updates own knowledge through inquiry and independent study		
2. Teaches staff utilizing past and present experience		
3. Assists others in evaluating the effectiveness of nursing care rendered		

Continued on following page

Preanesthesia Nursing Competency Level III	Comments/Goals	Competency Met Date and Initial
4. Proposes alternative for self-improvement		
C. Participates in Quality Improvement Activities		
1. Offers positive suggestions for identified problems and/or researchable problems		
2. Cooperates and follows through with research activities and/or planned change		

_____ has achieved Level III Senior Preanesthesia Nursing proficiency

_____   _____

Manager   Date

9

Advanced Pre Anesthesia Nurse

Level IV/Step 1

I. Provides Nursing Care to Patients with Alterations in Health Management
   A. Demonstrates autonomy in rendering care and in clinical decision-making
   B. Demonstrates competency in managing multiproblem nursing situations
II. Participates in Professional Growth and Development
   A. Monitors and maintains a therapeutic environment for staff and patients
   B. Acts as catalyst for change in the grooming process
   C. Participates in clinical education activities

Preanesthesia Nursing Knowledge Level IV/Step 1	Comments/Goals	Competency Met Date and Initial
I. Provides Nursing Care to Patients with Alterations in Health Management		
1. Formulates and describes own leadership style		
2. Describes own definition of risk-taking		
3. Describes patient care situation that indicates high-level clinical decision-making capabilities		
4. Analyzes and evaluates researchable data in relation to preanesthesia nursing care		
5. Compares this hospital's preanesthesia nursing practice to that of other hospitals		

Continued on following page

Preanesthesia Nursing Knowledge *Continued* Level IV/Step 1	Comments/Goals	Competency Met Date and Initial
II. Participates in Professional Growth and Development		
1. Describes own definition of a therapeutic recovery unit environment		
2. Proposes ways to maintain an atmosphere of open communication and trust		
3. Develops and describes own method of feedback and counseling		
4. Describes methods of conflict resolution		
5. Evaluates alternatives in peer grooming process		
6. Differentiates between androgogical and pedagogical teaching methods		
7. Discusses alternatives for teaching and learning		
8. Describes the preceptor role, indicating its value in the preanesthesia unit		

Continued on following page

Preanesthesia Nursing Competencies Level IV/Step 1	Comments/Goals	Competency Met Date and Initial
I. Provides Nursing Care to Patients with Alterations in Health Management		
A. Demonstrates Autonomy in Rendering Care and in Clinical Decision-Making		
1. Makes independent judgments and initiates follow through; seeks consultation appropriately		
2. Applies current nursing research findings to clinical practice		
3. Evaluates effectiveness of preanesthesia nursing care standards and nursing care rendered in relation to patient outcome		
4. Adjusts nursing care and clinical decisions based on predicted and observed patient outcome		
B. Demonstrates Competency in Managing Multiproblem Nursing Situations		
1. Judges qualitative situations involving multiple variables		
2. "Hones in" on accurate region of preventing problems		

Continued on following page

Preanesthesia Nursing Competencies *Continued* Level IV/Step 1	Comments/Goals	Competency Met Date and Initial
3. Predicts outcomes based on knowledge and clinical experience		
4. Manages routine standards, procedures, and guidelines effectively in the context of multiple-care needs		

Continued on following page

Preanesthesia Nursing Competencies *Continued* Level IV/Step 1	Comments/Goals	Competency Met Date and Initial
II. Participates in Professional Growth and Development		
A. Monitors and Maintains a Therapeutic Environment for Staff and Patients		
1. Anticipates potential problems and manages staff accordingly		
2. Plans for next-shift staffing needs, anticipating staffing needs for the next 24 hours		
3. Utilizes resources within the milieu to provide for problem-solving		
4. Creates an atmosphere of trust, confidence, and open communication		
5. Utilizes discretionary judgment in patient care assignments (correlates nursing skill level with patient activity)		
6. Independently takes charge or acts as a resource in emergency situations		
B. Acts as Catalyst for Change in the Grooming Process		
1. Initiates counseling on complex issues and communicates same to managers		

Continued on following page

Preanesthesia Nursing Competencies *Continued* Level IV/Step 1	Comments/Goals	Competency Met Date and Initial
2. Writes informative and ongoing anecdotal notes		
3. Follows through after counseling, as guided by manager		
C. Participates in Clinical Education Activities		
1. Updates own knowledge through self-motivated independent study; goes after learning experiences		
2. Assists others in evaluation of nursing care standards, nursing care rendered, and patient outcomes		
3. Shares information from various resources and current research for maintaining quality nursing care in a formal manner		
4. Participates in exploring nursing issues related to clinical practice		

Continued on following page

Preanesthesia Nursing Competencies *Continued* Level IV/Step 1	Comments/Goals	Competency Met Date and Initial
5. Collaborates with health care team members in evaluating and implementing planned change		
6. Acts as preceptor for nursing personnel, implementing clinical instruction based on mutual goals		

_____ has achieved Level IV/Step 1 Advanced Preanesthesia Nursing proficiency.

_____   _____
Manager   Date

Level IV/Step 2

I. Provides Nursing Care to Patients with Alterations in Health Management

    A. Effectively manages and coordinates complex and changing patients needs and staffing needs

II. Participates in Professional Growth and Development

    A. Participates in activities that contribute to development of a professional body of knowledge, with emphasis on the specialty of preanesthesia care

    B. Acts as agent of change in the grooming process

Preanesthesia Nursing Competencies Level IV/Step 2	Comments/Goals	Competency Met Date and Initial
I. Provides Nursing Care to Patients with Alterations in Health Management		
A. Effectively Manages and Coordinates Complex and Change Patient Needs and Staffing Needs		
1. Recognizes the needs of the entire unit at any given time and offers assistance, suggestions, and alternatives when needed		
2. Remains flexible within the organization of the unit, promptly recognizing changing needs, evaluating effectiveness of current plan, and altering the plan as necessary		
3. Takes risks based on secure and accurate judgments in both unit needs and patient care needs		

Continued on following page

Preanesthesia Nursing Competencies *Continued* Level IV/Step 2	Comments/Goals	Competency Met Date and Initial
II. Participates in Professional Growth and Development		
A. Participates in Activities that Contribute to the Development of a Professional Body of Knowledge, with Emphasis on the Speciality of Preanesthesia Care		
B. Acts as Agent of Change in the Grooming Process		
1. Creates an atmosphere that promotes evaluation of nursing care and nursing standards		
2. Takes a leadership role in assisting others to identify, evaluate, and maintain nursing standards of care		
3. Assists others in exploring educational opportunities to promote professional development		
4. Provides opportunities for other personnel to attain clinical knowledge and develop clinical skills		

Continued on following page

Preanesthesia Nursing Competencies *Continued* Level IV/Step 2	Comments/Goals	Competency Met Date and Initial
5. Facilitates behavior modification on an individual basis		
6. Follows through with the process of behavior modification on a long-term basis		
7. Assists others in goal-setting		
8. Participates in peer evaluation		

_____ has achieved Level IV/Step 2 Advanced Preanesthesia Nursing proficiency.

_____   _____

Manager   Date

PREANESTHESIA AND POSTANESTHESIA NURSING CLINICAL COMPETENCIES FOR PEDIATRIC CARE

10

Pediatric Competencies for the Level I Beginner Pre- and Post Anesthesia Nurse

I. Provides Nursing Care to Patients with Alterations in Health Care Management
  A. Demonstrates competency in caring for pediatric patients and their parents or guardians
II. Provides Nursing Care to Patients with Alterations in Activity-Exercise Patterns
  A. With minimal supervision, provides care to pediatric patients with respiratory dysfunction
  B. With minimal supervision, provides care to pediatric patients with alterations in fluid and/or blood volume

Beginner Pediatric Pre- & Postanesthesia Nursing Competencies Level I	Comments/Goals	Competency Met Date and Initial
I. Provides Nursing Care to Patients with Alterations in Health Care Management		
A. Demonstrates Competency in Caring for Pediatric Patients and Their Parents or Guardians		
1. Identifies major achievements according to Ericksen's five pediatric developmental stages		
2. Identifies motor and language skill development through infancy and childhood		
3. Initiates strategies that enhances the nurse-child relationship		
4. Recognizes five common childhood fears		
5. Devises strategies to deal with childhood fears, based on the developmental stages		
6. Initiates strategies that enhances the nurse-parent relationship		
7. Accurately administers drugs to the pediatric population:		

Continued on following page

Beginner Pediatric Pre- & Postanesthesia Nursing Competencies *Continued* Level I	Comments/Goals	Competency Met Date and Initial
a. Utilizes resources when administering antibiotics		
b. Calculates accurate dosage and dilution of all drugs		
c. Calculates accurate dosages for emergency drugs		
8. Demonstrates correct CPR for the infant and child		
9. Identifies internal and external factors that affect thermoregulation		
10. Initiates therapies to maintain temperature		

Beginner Pediatric Pre- & Postanesthesia Nursing Competencies *Continued* Level I	Comments/Goals	Competency Met Date and Initial
II. Provides Nursing Care to Patients with Alterations in Activity-Exercise Patterns		
A. With Minimal Supervision, Provides Care to Pediatric Patients with Respiratory Dysfunction		
1. Compare anatomical differences in the pediatric airway and thoracic cage to those of the adult		
2. Consistently ausculates or feels for air exchange with every respiratory assessment		
3. Effectively ventilates with ambu and mask		
B. With Minimal Supervision, Provides Care to Pediatric Patients with Alterations in Fluid and/or Blood Volume		
1. Compares differences in the pediatric fluid volumes to those of the adult		
2. Identifies three factors influencing pediatric hydration		
3. Calculates normal pediatric blood volume and percent lost during surgery		

Continued on following page

Beginner Pediatric Pre- & Postanesthesia Nursing Competencies *Continued* Level I	Comments/Goals	Competency Met Date and Initial
4. Identifies normal hematocrit and hemoglobin levels for the neonate, infant, and child		
5. Correctly administers blood products to the pediatric patient		

_____ has met the criteria of the Pediatric Competencies for the Level I Beginner Pre- and Post Anesthesia Nurse.

_____   _____

Manager   Date

11

Pediatric Competencies for the Level II Pre- and Post Anesthesia Nurse

I. Provides Nursing Care to Patients with Alterations in Health Management

    A. Demonstrates competency in caring for complex pediatric patients and their parents or guardians

    B. Provides coordination of pediatric patient care activities

II. Provides Nursing Care to Patients with Alterations in Activity-Exercise Patterns

    A. Provides care to pediatric patients with complex respiratory dysfunction

III. Provides Nursing Care to Patients with Alterations in Cognitive and Perceptual Patterns

    A. Independently cares for pediatric patients with alterations in level of consciousness

Pediatric Pre- & Postanesthesia Nursing Competencies Level II	Comments/Goals	Competency Met Date and Initial
I. Provides Nursing Care to Patients with Alterations in Health Management		
A. Demonstrates Competency in Caring for Complex Pediatric Patients		
1. Demonstrates accurate nursing care for the infant and child requiring invasive lines		
2. Reacts efficiently and effectively in pediatric emergency situations		
3. Discusses concepts related to the most commonly seen postanesthesia pediatric surgical patients:		
a. Ophthalmic		
b. Otolaryngologic		
c. Neurosurgical		
d. Orthopedic		

Continued on following page

Pediatric Pre- & Postanesthesia Nursing Competencies *Continued* Level II	Comments/Goals	Competency Met Date and Initial
e. Gastrointestinal		
f. Urologic		
B. Provides Coordination of Pediatric Patient Care Activities		
1. Identifies, implements, and evaluates the plan of care for all types of postanesthesia *pediatric* patients (noncomplex, extended-care, complex, unstable complex)		
2. Initiates respiratory care and implements nursing measures to correct hypoxia and/or hypercarbia in the pediatric patient		
3. Anticipates use, pediatric dosage, and pediatric response to bronchodilators		
4. Prepares for pediatric endotracheal intubation		
5. Initiates appropriate nursing measures for the intubated infant or child		

Continued on following page

Pediatric Pre- & Postanesthesia Nursing Competencies *Continued* Level II	Comments/Goals	Competency Met Date and Initial
III. Provides Nursing Care to Patients with Alterations in Cognitive and Perceptual Patterns		
A. Independently Cares for Pediatric Patients with Alterations in Level of Consciousness		
1. Identifies commonly used anesthetics for the pediatric population		
2. Initiates appropriate nursing interventions to prevent and/or treat postanesthesia pediatric complications		
3. Provides safety measures during emergence from anesthesia		
4. Anticipates the need for pain relief on emergence from anesthesia		

_____ has met the criteria of the Pediatric Competencies for the Level II Pre- and Post Anesthesia Nurse.

_____   _____

Manager   Date

Bibliography

Anesthesia

Cote CJ et al (1992) *A Practice of Anesthesia for Infants & Children*. (2nd Ed). Philadelphia: WB Saunders.

Longnecher DE, and Murphy FL (Eds) (1992) *Dripps/Eckenhoff/Vandam: Introduction to Anesthesia*. Philadelphia: WB Saunders.

Wetchler BV (Ed) (1991) *Anesthesia for Ambulatory Surgery* (2nd Ed). Philadelphia: JB Lippincott.

Postanesthesia Nursing

Burden N (1993) *Ambulatory Surgical Nursing*. Philadelphia: WB Saunders.

Drain CB (1994) *The Post Anesthesia Care Unit (PACU): A Critical Care Approach to Post Anesthesia Nursing*. Philadelphia: WB Saunders.

Gruendemann B (1987) *Alexander's Care of the Patient in Surgery* (8th Ed). St. Louis: Mosby-Year Book.

Hathaway RG (1988) *Nursing Care of the Critically Ill Surgical Patient*. Rockville, MD: Aspen Publishers.

Jacobsen WK (Ed) (1992) *Manual of Post Anesthesia Care*. Philadelphia: WB Saunders.

Litwack K (1990) *Post Anesthesia Care Nursing*. St Louis: Mosby-Year Book.

Litwack K (Ed) (1995) *Core Curriculum for Post Anesthesia Nursing Practice* (3rd ed) Philadelphia: WB Saunders.

Luczun ME (1987) *Handbook of Post Anesthesia Nursing*. Rockville, MD: Aspen Publishers.

Physician's Desk Reference (1993).

Shannon MT and Wilson BA (1993) *Govoni & Hayes: Drugs and Nursing Implications* (7th ed). East Norwalk, CT: Appleton & Lange.

Vender J and Spiess B (1992) *Post Anesthesia Care*. Philadelphia: WB Saunders.

Respiratory

Huddleston VB (1990) Pulmonary problems. *Crit Care Nurs Clin North Am 2*(4), 527–536.

Schultheis AH (1989) When and how to extubate in the recovery room. *Am J Nurs* *89*(8), 1040–1047.

Shapiro BA, Harrison RA, Cane RD, and Templin R (1989) *Clinical Application of Blood Gases* (4th Ed). Chicago: Year Book Medical Publishers.

Cardiovascular

Grauer K and Cavallars D (1987) *ACLS Certification Preparation and Comprehensive Review*. St. Louis: Mosby-Year Book.

Strong AG (1991) Nursing management of postoperative dysrhythmia. *Crit Care Nurs Clin North Am* *3*(4), 709–715.

Walraven G (1992) *Basic Arrhythmias* (3rd Ed). Englewood Cliffs, NJ: Prentice-Hall.

Wiederhold R (1988) *Electrocardiography: The Monitoring Lead*. Philadelphia: WB Saunders.

Pediatric

Jaffee M (1993) *Pediatric Nursing Care Plans*. El Paso, TX: Skidmore-Roth.

Wilson TA and Graves SA (1990) Pediatric considerations in a general postanesthesia care unit. *J Post Anesth Nurs* *5*(1), 16–24.

Wong DL (1993) *Whaley and Wong's Essentials of Pediatric Nursing* (4th ed). St. Louis: Mosby-Year Book.

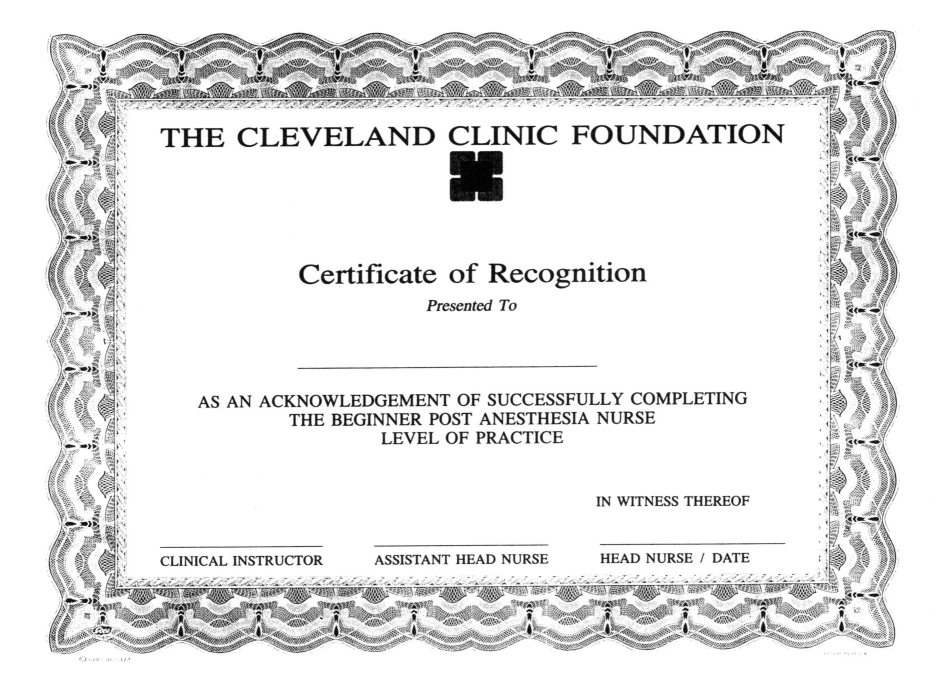

THE CLEVELAND CLINIC FOUNDATION

Certificate of Recognition

Presented To

_____

AS AN ACKNOWLEDGEMENT OF SUCCESSFULLY COMPLETING
THE BEGINNER POST ANESTHESIA NURSE
LEVEL OF PRACTICE

IN WITNESS THEREOF

_____   _____   _____

CLINICAL INSTRUCTOR   ASSISTANT HEAD NURSE   HEAD NURSE / DATE

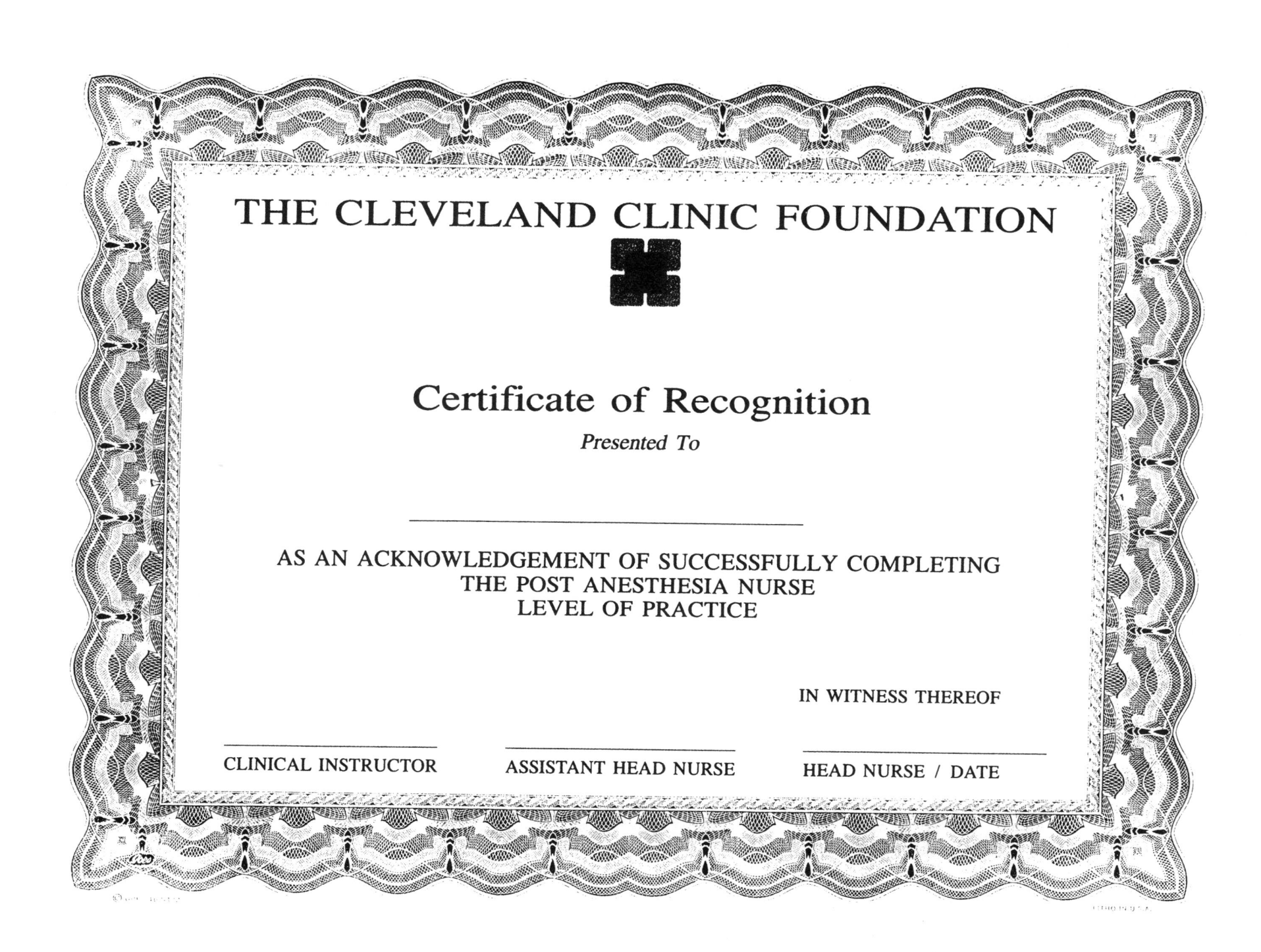

THE CLEVELAND CLINIC FOUNDATION

Certificate of Recognition

Presented To

_____

AS AN ACKNOWLEDGEMENT OF SUCCESSFULLY COMPLETING
THE POST ANESTHESIA NURSE
LEVEL OF PRACTICE

IN WITNESS THEREOF

_____   _____   _____
CLINICAL INSTRUCTOR   ASSISTANT HEAD NURSE   HEAD NURSE / DATE

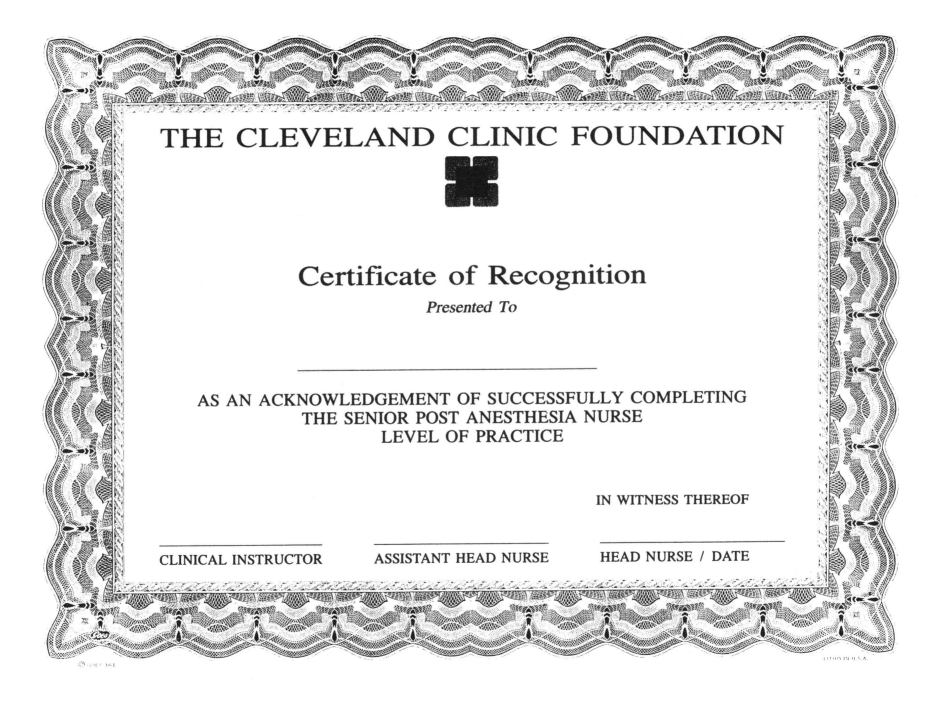

THE CLEVELAND CLINIC FOUNDATION

Certificate of Recognition

Presented To

_____

AS AN ACKNOWLEDGEMENT OF SUCCESSFULLY COMPLETING
THE SENIOR POST ANESTHESIA NURSE
LEVEL OF PRACTICE

IN WITNESS THEREOF

_____   _____   _____
CLINICAL INSTRUCTOR   ASSISTANT HEAD NURSE   HEAD NURSE / DATE

LITHO IN U.S.A.

THE CLEVELAND CLINIC FOUNDATION

Certificate of Recognition

Presented To

_____

AS AN ACKNOWLEDGEMENT OF SUCCESSFULLY COMPLETING
THE ADVANCED POST ANESTHESIA NURSE
LEVEL OF PRACTICE

IN WITNESS THEREOF

_____   _____   _____

CLINICAL INSTRUCTOR   ASSISTANT HEAD NURSE   HEAD NURSE / DATE

Index